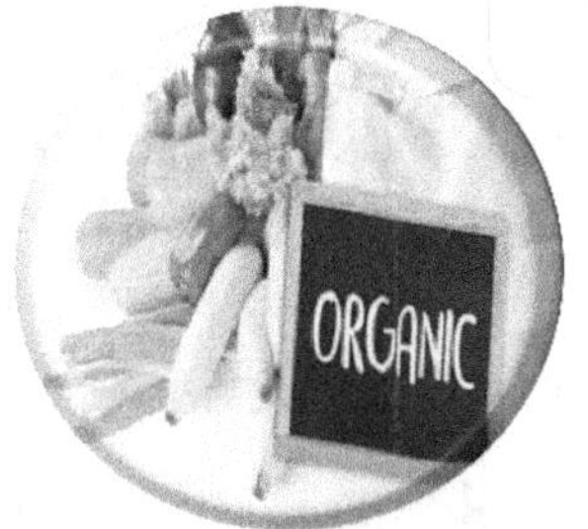

ALKALINE REMEDIES

AGAINST CANCER

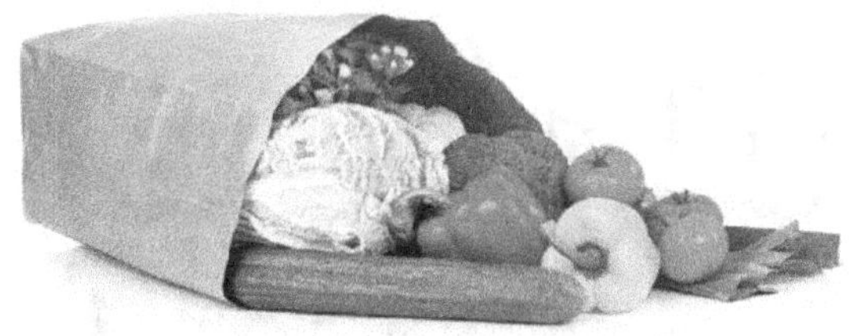

Quick and easy 30 Nourishing Plant-Based Smoothies for Cancer Prevention

Dr. VIVIAN GREENE

COPYRIGHT © 2024 DR. VIVIAN GREENE

Please scan the QR code to access additional books authored by Dr. Vivian Greene

TABLE OF CONTENTS

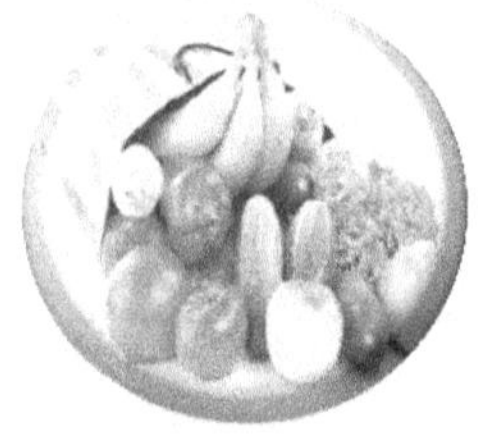

Introduction

In a society where being well is the greatest asset, finding treatments to break the unbreakable hold of cancer takes center stage. An engaging investigation of the relationship between holistic nutrition and the prevention of cancer may be found in "Alkaline Remedies Against Cancer: Quick and Easy 30 Nourishing Plant-Based Smoothies for Cancer Prevention". Discover in these pages the revolutionary power of alkaline-rich therapies and their tremendous influence on both preventing and impeding the progression of cancer.

This book celebrates the nutritious core of plant-based smoothies as a potent weapon in the fight against this tough foe, attesting to the healing power of nature's abundance. Discover the essence of alkalinity, the power of thoughtfully chosen ingredients, and the joy of creating 30 reviving smoothie recipes that are all vivid combinations of flavor, health, and hope.

Take a trip via these pages that reveal the union of scientific research and culinary talent, allowing you to enjoy the flavors of wellness and strengthen your body's resistance to cancer.

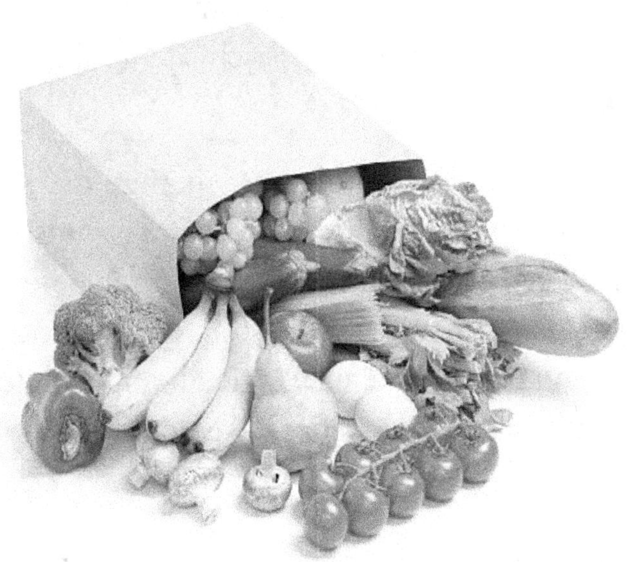

Understanding Alkaline Remedies for Cancer Prevention

It is important to comprehend the complex connection between pH balance and the body's ability to fend off malignant development in order to comprehend alkaline treatments for cancer prevention. The idea behind alkaline treatments is that an alkaline environment inside the body makes it difficult for cancer cells to proliferate. This idea encourages research into how food and drink affect the pH levels of the body and highlights the need to include more alkaline-rich items in one's diet.

Research indicates that an alkaline diet, rich in fruits, vegetables, and certain nuts and seeds, supports the body's natural defenses against cancer in addition to helping to maintain a pH balance. The alkaline strategy emphasizes how critical it is to cut down on acidic foods, sweets, and processed meat as they might cause the body's pH to become more acidic, which could encourage the growth of cancer.

Gaining knowledge about alkaline treatments for cancer prevention is a liberating experience that emphasizes the role that dietary changes may play in strengthening the body's defenses against the advent of this deadly illness.

The Power of Plant-Based Smoothies in Fighting Cancer

Plant-based smoothies are a powerful weapon against cancer because they are packed with nutrients, antioxidants, and bioactive substances that come from nature's abundance. These colorful mixtures provide targeted administration of vital vitamins, minerals, and phytochemicals that promote a cellular environment that inhibits the growth of cancerous cells.

Smoothies made with plant-based ingredients are a powerful combination of fruits, vegetables, leafy greens, and seeds, each of which has specific anti-cancer benefits. Rich in antioxidants such as beta-carotene, vitamin C, and flavonoids, these smoothies reduce oxidative stress and cellular damage caused by damaging free radicals, which in turn is a trigger for the development of cancer.

The high fiber content of plant-based components supports healthy gut microbiota, assists in detoxification, and enhances the body's immunological response against cancer.

The ease with which these components may be combined to create delicious, approachable drinks improves their availability and assimilation into regular eating routines, supporting people in their fight against cancer. Using plant-based smoothies as a means of boosting immunity, promoting general health, and maybe delaying the development of cancer is a tasty and nutritious approach.

Section I

ALKALINE REMEDIES AND

CANCER PREVENTION

By focusing on the pH levels of the body, alkaline treatments are essential in the fight against cancer because they create an environment that hinders the formation and multiplication of cancer cells. The key to alkalinity is to keep your pH in check and err on the side of alkalinity, which is thought to inhibit the growth and survival of malignant cells.

Studies show that eating a diet high in fruits, vegetables, nuts, and seeds—which are mostly alkaline—helps the body maintain a healthy pH balance. This dietary strategy aims to reduce excessive acidity, which may accelerate the development of cancer. People try to reset their internal pH by consuming more alkaline-forming foods and drinks and less acidic substances such as processed meals, sweets, and certain animal products. This creates an environment that inhibits the formation of cancer.

Although more thorough research is needed to determine the precise effect of alkaline treatments on cancer prevention, adopting an alkaline-focused lifestyle offers a potential way to strengthen the body's defenses against cancer and improve general health and well-being.

Exploring Alkalinity and its Role in Cancer Prevention

Investigating alkalinity reveals an intriguing area in the field of cancer prevention by examining the complex equilibrium of pH levels in the human body and its possible influence on impeding the growth of cancer. The idea is to keep the pH balance as close to neutral as possible, preferably slightly alkaline since this is thought to inhibit the development and spread of cancer cells.

Given that cancer cells often grow in acidic environments, research indicates that an alkaline environment may slow the spread of the disease. Therefore, a proactive strategy for strengthening the body's natural defensive systems is to comprehend and promote alkalinity via dietary and lifestyle choices.

Alkalinity research focuses on reducing acidic components found in processed diets, sweets, and certain animal products while increasing alkaline-forming foods including fruits, nuts, and seeds. This sophisticated knowledge emphasizes how dietary modifications may affect the body's pH balance and perhaps reduce the internal milieu that supports the growth of cancer.

Examining alkalinity in cancer prevention offers an intriguing convergence of nutritional science and holistic well-being, providing people with a proactive approach to maintaining their health and perhaps reducing the conditions that lead to the development and spread of cancer.

Key Alkaline Ingredients for Combatting Cancer

Important alkaline components are powerful partners in the fight against cancer because of their ability to create an alkaline environment in the body and maybe stop the formation of malignant cells. These components serve as the foundation of an anti-cancer diet since they are abundant in vital nutrients and have alkalizing qualities.

Leafy Greens: Rich in antioxidants and chlorophyll, varieties such as spinach, kale, and Swiss chard help with detoxification and strengthen the immune system to fight cancer.

Cruciferous Vegetables: Brussels sprouts, cauliflower, and broccoli are rich in sulfur-containing phytochemicals and compounds that support cancer prevention and detoxification.

Citrus Fruits: Despite their acidic flavor, lemons, oranges, and grapefruits help to create an alkaline environment in the body by metabolizing to alkaline byproducts.

Berries: Packed with anthocyanins, which are powerful antioxidants, berries like raspberries and blueberries help to fight oxidative stress and may even lower the risk of cancer.

Almonds and Seeds: Rich in fiber and vital fatty acids, almonds, flaxseeds, and chia seeds are alkaline-forming foods that promote general health and may even prevent the growth of cancer.

Avocado: Rich in nutrients and alkaline-forming, this fruit provides monounsaturated fats, vitamins, and antioxidants that help maintain a pH equilibrium.

By adding these essential alkaline foods to one's diet, one may take a calculated approach to creating an alkaline environment that may slow the spread of cancer and improve general health and well-being.

Section II

NOURISHING PLANT-BASED

SMOOTHIES

Nourishing plant-based smoothies epitomize a vibrant fusion of health and flavor, offering a delightful gateway to wellness through the consumption of nature's bounty. These beverages, crafted from an assortment of plant-derived ingredients, stand as a testament to the nourishing potential of fruits, vegetables, leafy greens, nuts, and seeds.

The essence of these smoothies lies not only in their refreshing taste but also in their nutrient density. Blending an array of wholesome components unlocks a treasure trove of vitamins, minerals, antioxidants, and phytochemicals. This powerful concoction not only satisfies the palate but also fuels the body with essential nutrients, fostering vitality and fortifying the immune system.

The versatility of plant-based smoothies allows for endless creativity, enabling individuals to tailor blends to their preferences and nutritional needs. Whether concocting a green elixir packed with kale, spinach, and avocado or a vibrant berry medley infused with antioxidants, each sip represents a potent amalgamation of healthful elements.

These smoothies transcend mere refreshment; they serve as an accessible and delectable means of incorporating an abundance of plant-based goodness into one's daily routine. Embracing nourishing plant-based smoothies signifies an enjoyable pathway to wellness, promoting optimal health while savoring the abundance of flavors nature has to offer.

Basics of Crafting Nourishing Smoothies

Making healthy smoothies starts with a base of creativity and simplicity, which provides a canvas on which to combine a variety of healthful ingredients to create a delicious and nutrient-dense drink.

The first step in selecting ingredients is to gather a variety of fruits, vegetables, leafy greens, nuts, seeds, and liquid bases such as coconut water, nut milk, and water. When possible, choose organic, fresh produce to optimize its nutritional value.

Combining sweet fruits like bananas or berries with vegetables or leafy greens may help achieve a balance of textures and tastes. Use foods like Greek yogurt or avocados to provide creamy textures. For a crunchier texture and a boost of protein and good fats, add nuts or seeds.

Increasing Nutritional Density: To increase nutritional content, use superfoods such as maca powder, spirulina, chia seeds, and flaxseeds. These supplements provide important minerals, vitamins, antioxidants, and health-promoting substances.

Blending Techniques: To guarantee correct blending and prevent overtaxing the equipment, layer items in the blender. To produce a smooth consistency, start with liquids, then add softer foods, leafy greens, frozen fruits, and ice or frozen goods.

Customizing and Trying New Things: Modify ingredient amounts to accommodate dietary requirements and personal taste preferences. Try blending various ingredients, tastes, and textures to create interesting and delightful concoctions.

Learning the fundamentals of making nutritious smoothies enables people to make customized blends that stimulate taste senses and provide a concentrated dosage of vital nutrients that promote general health and well-being.

Smoothies as a Convenient Tool for Cancer Prevention

Smoothies are an easily incorporated approach to adding a multitude of anti-cancer nutrients to one's daily routine, making them a useful and adaptable weapon in the battle against cancer.

Nutrient Density: Made from a wide variety of fruits, vegetables, and other plant-based components, these blended drinks provide a potent punch of vital vitamins, minerals, antioxidants, and phytochemicals. This targeted dietary intake helps the body's defenses against oxidative stress and the formation of malignant cells.

Alkalizing Potential: Drinks made with alkaline-forming components help the body's pH stay in equilibrium. These drinks may prevent the growth of cancer by lowering acidity and promoting an alkaline environment.

Ease of Consumption: Smoothies are a quick and effective way to get a range of foods that prevent cancer in one serving. People who lead hectic lives or struggle to consume solid meals because of sickness or therapy may especially benefit from this accessibility.

Customization for Particular Needs: Smoothies may be made to meet the nutritional needs and tastes of each person. Including foods that are known to have anti-cancer qualities, including berries, nuts, seeds, and leafy greens, allows for a customized approach to nutrition-based cancer prevention.

Smoothies are an easy way for people to increase their consumption of nutrients that fight cancer, which may promote general health and perhaps lower the chance of developing cancer. Smoothies play an important part in the proactive pursuit of cancer prevention techniques, as shown by this easy and fun approach to nutrition.

Section III

30 Quick and Easy Plant-Based Smoothie Recipes

Green Leafy Elixirs: Recipes 1-10

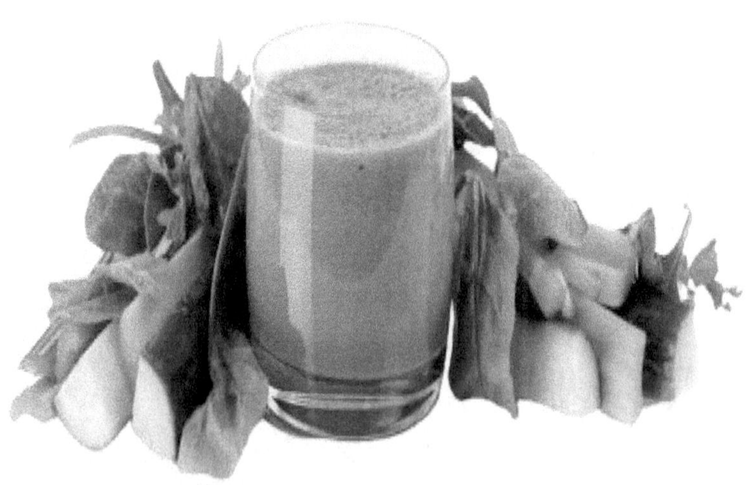

RECIPE 1: "VIBRANT SPINACH BOOST"

INGREDIENTS

1. 1 cup fresh spinach leaves
2. 1 ripe banana
3. 1/2 cup pineapple chunks
4. 1 tablespoon chia seeds
5. 1 cup coconut water

INSTRUCTIONS

1. Blend spinach, banana, pineapple, and chia seeds until smooth.
2. Add coconut water gradually for desired consistency.
3. Serve chilled and enjoy!

NUTRITION PER SERVING

- ❖ *Calories: 180*
- ❖ *Protein: 4g*
- ❖ *Fiber: 8g*
- ❖ *Vitamin C: 45% DV*
- ❖ *Iron: 15% DV*

Recipe 2: "Kale Power Punch"

INGREDIENTS

1. 1 cup kale leaves (stems removed)
2. 1 green apple (cored and chopped)
3. 1/2 cucumber (peeled and sliced)
4. Juice of 1 lemon
5. 1 tablespoon hemp seeds
6. 1 cup almond milk

INSTRUCTIONS

1. Combine kale, apple, cucumber, lemon juice, and hemp seeds in a blender.
2. Add almond milk gradually and blend until smooth.
3. Pour into a glass and enjoy the freshness!

NUTRITION PER SERVING

- ❖ *Calories: 150*
- ❖ *Protein: 5g*
- ❖ *Fiber: 6g*
- ❖ *Vitamin A: 200% DV*
- ❖ *Vitamin K: 250% DV*

RECIPE 3: "REFRESHING GREEN GODDESS"

INGREDIENTS

1. 1 cup baby spinach
2. 1/2 cup green grapes
3. 1/2 ripe pear
4. 1/2 avocado
5. 1 tablespoon fresh mint leaves
6. 1/2 cup coconut water

INSTRUCTIONS

1. Blend spinach, grapes, pear, avocado, and mint until creamy.
2. Gradually add coconut water for desired consistency.
3. Pour into a glass, garnish with mint, and savor the refreshment!

NUTRITION PER SERVING

❖ *Calories: 200*
❖ *Protein: 3g*
❖ *Fiber: 9g*
❖ *Vitamin E: 15% DV*
❖ *Potassium: 20% DV*

Recipe 4: "Tropical Kale Fusion"

INGREDIENTS

1. 1 cup kale leaves
2. 1/2 cup frozen mango chunks
3. 1/2 cup pineapple chunks
4. 1 tablespoon flaxseeds
5. 1 cup orange juice

INSTRUCTIONS

1. Blend kale, mango, pineapple, and flaxseeds until smooth.
2. Gradually pour in orange juice while blending to reach desired consistency.
3. Pour into a glass, feel the tropical vibes, and enjoy!

NUTRITION PER SERVING

- ❖ *Calories: 190*
- ❖ *Protein: 4g*
- ❖ *Fiber: 7g*
- ❖ *Vitamin C: 160% DV*
- ❖ *Vitamin A: 90% DV*

RECIPE 5: "SPINACH-BERRY BLISS"

INGREDIENTS

1. 1 cup fresh spinach
2. 1/2 cup strawberries
3. 1/2 cup blueberries
4. 1 tablespoon almond butter
5. 1 cup unsweetened almond milk

INSTRUCTIONS

1. Blend spinach, strawberries, blueberries, and almond butter until creamy.
2. Add almond milk gradually for desired consistency.
3. Pour into a glass, relish the berry goodness, and embrace the bliss!

NUTRITION PER SERVING

- *Calories: 170*
- *Protein: 5g*
- *Fiber: 8g*
- *Vitamin K: 110% DV*
- *Manganese: 25% DV*

RECIPE 6: "SUPERCHARGED GREEN SMOOTHIE"

INGREDIENTS

1. 1 cup Swiss chard leaves
2. 1/2 ripe banana
3. 1/2 cup pineapple chunks
4. 1 tablespoon spirulina powder
5. 1 cup water or coconut water

INSTRUCTIONS

1. Blend Swiss chard, banana, pineapple, and spirulina until smooth.
2. Add water or coconut water gradually for desired consistency.
3. Pour into a glass, feel the nutrient boost, and relish the goodness!

NUTRITION PER SERVING

- *Calories: 160*
- *Protein: 5g*
- *Fiber: 6g*
- *Iron: 20% DV*
- *Vitamin C: 70% DV*

RECIPE 7: "AVOCADO-KALE DREAM"

INGREDIENTS

1. 1 cup kale leaves
2. 1/2 ripe avocado
3. 1/2 cucumber
4. 1/2 green apple
5. Juice of 1 lime
6. 1 cup coconut water

INSTRUCTIONS

1. Blend kale, avocado, cucumber, apple, and lime juice until creamy.
2. Gradually add coconut water for desired consistency.
3. Pour into a glass, enjoy the creamy texture, and savor the green dream!

NUTRITION PER SERVING

- *Calories: 180*
- *Protein: 4g*
- *Fiber: 9g*
- *Vitamin K: 200% DV*
- *Potassium: 25% DV*

RECIPE 8: "SAVORY SPINACH DELIGHT"

INGREDIENTS

1. 1 cup fresh spinach leaves
2. 1/2 cup cooked quinoa (cooled)
3. 1/2 cucumber (peeled and chopped)
4. 1/4 avocado
5. 1 tablespoon fresh parsley
6. 1 cup unsweetened almond milk

INSTRUCTIONS

1. Blend spinach, quinoa, cucumber, avocado, parsley, and almond milk until smooth.
2. Adjust almond milk for desired consistency.
3. Pour into a glass, relish the unique blend, and enjoy the savory delight!

NUTRITION PER SERVING

- ❖ *Calories: 200*
- ❖ *Protein: 6g*
- ❖ *Fiber: 8g*
- ❖ *Vitamin E: 25% DV*
- ❖ *Magnesium: 20% DV*

RECIPE 9: "MINTY GREEN REVITALIZER"

INGREDIENTS

1. 1 cup baby spinach
2. 1/2 cup fresh mint leaves
3. 1/2 cucumber
4. 1/2 green apple
5. 1 tablespoon honey or agave syrup
6. 1 cup coconut water

INSTRUCTIONS

1. Blend spinach, mint, cucumber, apple, and sweetener until well combined.
2. Gradually add coconut water for desired consistency.
3. Pour into a glass, feel the refreshing mint, and revitalize your day!

NUTRITION PER SERVING

- *Calories: 150*
- *Protein: 3g*
- *Fiber: 6g*
- *Vitamin A: 80% DV*
- *Manganese: 15% DV*

RECIPE 10: "CHIA-KALE ENERGIZER"

INGREDIENTS

1. 1 cup kale leaves
2. 1/2 cup pineapple chunks
3. 1 tablespoon chia seeds
4. 1 tablespoon almond butter
5. 1 cup unsweetened almond milk

INSTRUCTIONS

1. Blend kale, pineapple, chia seeds, almond butter, and almond milk until smooth.
2. Adjust almond milk for desired thickness.
3. Pour into a glass, feel the energy boost, and savor the nutrient-packed goodness!

NUTRITION PER SERVING

- *Calories: 180*
- *Protein: 5g*
- *Fiber: 9g*
- *Vitamin C: 100% DV*
- *Calcium: 25% DV*

Berry Blasts: Recipes 11-20

RECIPE 11: BERRY BURST DELIGHT

INGREDIENTS

1. 1 cup mixed berries (strawberries, blueberries, raspberries)
2. 1 ripe banana
3. 1/2 cup spinach leaves
4. 1 tablespoon chia seeds
5. 1 cup almond milk

INSTRUCTIONS

1. Blend mixed berries, banana, spinach, chia seeds, and almond milk until smooth.
2. Pour into a glass and serve fresh.

NUTRITION PER SERVING

- ❖ *Calories: 180*
- ❖ *Carbohydrates: 35g*
- ❖ *Fiber: 10g*
- ❖ *Protein: 5g*
- ❖ *Fat: 4g*

RECIPE 12: RASPBERRY ZING SMOOTHIE

INGREDIENTS

1. 1 cup raspberries
2. 1/2 cup pineapple chunks
3. 1/2 cup coconut water
4. 1 tablespoon hemp seeds
5. Handful of kale

INSTRUCTIONS

1. Combine raspberries, pineapple, coconut water, hemp seeds, and kale in a blender.
2. Blend until creamy and serve immediately.

NUTRITION PER SERVING

- ❖ *Calories: 160*
- ❖ *Carbohydrates: 28g*
- ❖ *Fiber: 9g*
- ❖ *Protein: 6g*
- ❖ *Fat: 4g*

RECIPE 13: BLUEBERRY BLISS ELIXIR

INGREDIENTS

1. 1 cup blueberries
2. 1/2 cup Greek yogurt
3. 1 tablespoon almond butter
4. 1 teaspoon honey (optional)
5. 1/2 cup water or coconut water

INSTRUCTIONS

1. Blend blueberries, Greek yogurt, almond butter, honey, and water until well combined.
2. Pour into a glass and enjoy!

NUTRITION PER SERVING

- ❖ *Calories: 220*
- ❖ *Carbohydrates: 25g*
- ❖ *Fiber: 6g*
- ❖ *Protein: 12g*
- ❖ *Fat: 9g*

RECIPE 14: STRAWBERRY-KIWI MEDLEY

INGREDIENTS

1. 1 cup strawberries, hulled
2. 2 kiwis, peeled and sliced
3. 1/2 cup orange juice
4. Handful of spinach
5. 1 tablespoon flaxseeds

INSTRUCTIONS

1. Blend strawberries, kiwis, orange juice, spinach, and flaxseeds until smooth.
2. Pour into a glass and enjoy this refreshing blend.

NUTRITION PER SERVING

- ❖ *Calories: 150*
- ❖ *Carbohydrates: 35g*
- ❖ *Fiber: 8g*
- ❖ *Protein: 4g*
- ❖ *Fat: 3g*

RECIPE 15: BLACKBERRY BANANA BLISS

INGREDIENTS

1. 1 cup blackberries
2. 1 ripe banana
3. 1/2 cup almond milk
4. 1 tablespoon honey or maple syrup (optional)
5. Handful of kale or spinach

INSTRUCTIONS

1. Blend blackberries, banana, almond milk, sweetener (if using), and greens until creamy.
2. Pour into a glass and savor the vibrant flavors.

NUTRITION PER SERVING

- ❖ *Calories: 190*
- ❖ *Carbohydrates: 45g*
- ❖ *Fiber: 12g*
- ❖ *Protein: 5g*
- ❖ *Fat: 2g*

RECIPE 16: CRANBERRY-ORANGE ZEST

INGREDIENTS

1. 1/2 cup cranberries (fresh or frozen)
2. Juice of 1 orange
3. 1/2 cup coconut water
4. 1 tablespoon pumpkin seeds
5. 1 small carrot, chopped

INSTRUCTIONS

1. Blend cranberries, orange juice, coconut water, pumpkin seeds, and carrot until smooth.
2. Pour into a glass and relish the tangy-sweet goodness.

NUTRITION PER SERVING

- ❖ *Calories: 140*
- ❖ *Carbohydrates: 30g*
- ❖ *Fiber: 7g*
- ❖ *Protein: 4g*
- ❖ *Fat: 3g*

RECIPE 17: MIXED BERRY ANTIOXIDANT FUSION

INGREDIENTS

1. 1/2 cup mixed berries (strawberries, blueberries, blackberries)
2. 1/2 cup pomegranate juice
3. 1/2 cup Greek yogurt (or dairy-free alternative)
4. 1 tablespoon almond butter
5. Handful of spinach or kale

INSTRUCTIONS

1. Blend mixed berries, pomegranate juice, Greek yogurt, almond butter, and greens until well combined.
2. Pour into a glass and revel in the antioxidant-rich blend.

NUTRITION PER SERVING

- ❖ *Calories: 220*
- ❖ *Carbohydrates: 30g*
- ❖ *Fiber: 8g*
- ❖ *Protein: 12g*
- ❖ *Fat: 7g*

RECIPE 18: TROPICAL BERRY BREEZE

INGREDIENTS

1. 1/2 cup pineapple chunks
2. 1/2 cup mango chunks
3. 1/2 cup mixed berries (your choice)
4. 1/2 cup coconut water or almond milk
5. 1 tablespoon shredded coconut (optional)

INSTRUCTIONS

1. Blend pineapple, mango, mixed berries, and liquid until smooth.
2. Garnish with shredded coconut if desired and enjoy this tropical delight

NUTRITION PER SERVING

- *Calories: 180*
- *Carbohydrates: 40g*
- *Fiber: 8g*
- *Protein: 3g*
- *Fat: 2g*

RECIPE 19: CHERRY-ALMOND DREAM

INGREDIENTS

1. 1 cup cherries, pitted
2. 1/4 cup almonds (or almond butter)
3. 1/2 cup almond milk
4. 1 tablespoon honey or agave syrup (optional)
5. Handful of spinach or kale

INSTRUCTIONS

1. Blend cherries, almonds, almond milk, sweetener (if using), and greens until creamy.
2. Pour into a glass and savor the rich, nutty flavor.

NUTRITION PER SERVING

- *Calories: 250*
- *Carbohydrates: 30g*
- *Fiber: 6g*
- *Protein: 8g*
- *Fat: 12g*

RECIPE 20: RASPBERRY-COCONUT REFRESHER

INGREDIENTS

1. 1 cup raspberries
2. 1/2 cup coconut milk
3. 1/2 cup vanilla yogurt (or dairy-free alternative)
4. 1 tablespoon shredded coconut
5. Handful of baby spinach

INSTRUCTIONS

1. Blend raspberries, coconut milk, vanilla yogurt, shredded coconut, and spinach until well combined.
2. Pour into a glass, garnish with additional shredded coconut, and enjoy this tropical delight.

NUTRITION PER SERVING

- ❖ *Calories: 200*
- ❖ *Carbohydrates: 25g*
- ❖ *Fiber: 9g*
- ❖ *Protein: 6g*
- ❖ *Fat: 10g*

Tropical Treasures: Recipes 21-30

RECIPE 21: PINEAPPLE MANGO BLISS

INGREDIENTS

1. 1 cup chopped pineapple
2. 1 ripe mango, diced
3. 1 banana
4. 1/2 cup coconut water
5. Handful of spinach (optional)
6. Ice cubes (optional)

INSTRUCTIONS

1. Add pineapple, mango, banana, coconut water, and spinach to a blender.
2. Blend until smooth.
3. Add ice cubes for a cooler texture, if desired.
4. Pour into a glass and enjoy the tropical delight!

NUTRITION PER SERVING

- *Calories: 180*
- *Carbohydrates: 45g*
- *Fiber: 6g*
- *Protein: 3g*
- *Fat: 1g*

RECIPE 22: PASSIONFRUIT PAPAYA DREAM

INGREDIENTS

1. 1 ripe papaya, seeded and cubed
2. Pulp from 2 passionfruits
3. 1/2 cup plain Greek yogurt (or dairy-free yogurt)
4. 1 tablespoon honey or agave syrup (optional)
5. 1/2 cup almond milk
6. Ice cubes

INSTRUCTIONS

1. Blend papaya, passionfruit pulp, Greek yogurt, honey/agave syrup, and almond milk until smooth.
2. Add ice cubes for a frosty consistency.
3. Serve chilled in a glass and savor the tropical flavors!

NUTRITION PER SERVING

- *Calories: 210*
- *Carbohydrates: 40g*
- *Fiber: 5g*
- *Protein: 8g*
- *Fat: 4g*

RECIPE 23: KIWI COCONUT CRUSH

INGREDIENTS

1. 2 ripe kiwis, peeled and sliced
2. 1/2 cup coconut milk
3. 1/2 cup pineapple chunks
4. Handful of baby spinach
5. 1 tablespoon chia seeds (optional)
6. Ice cubes

INSTRUCTIONS

1. Blend kiwis, coconut milk, pineapple chunks, baby spinach, and chia seeds until smooth.
2. Add ice cubes for a cooler texture, if desired.
3. Pour into a glass and relish the refreshing blend!

NUTRITION PER SERVING

- ❖ *Calories: 220*
- ❖ *Carbohydrates: 30g*
- ❖ *Fiber: 8g*
- ❖ *Protein: 4g*
- ❖ *Fat: 10g*

Recipe 24: Guava Banana Tango

INGREDIENTS

1. 1 ripe guava, seeded and diced
2. 1 ripe banana
3. 1/2 cup orange juice
4. 1/2 cup unsweetened coconut water
5. Handful of kale leaves
6. Ice cubes

INSTRUCTIONS

1. Blend guava, banana, orange juice, coconut water, and kale leaves until creamy.
2. Incorporate ice cubes for a cooler, smoother consistency.
3. Serve chilled and revel in the tropical twist!

NUTRITION PER SERVING

- *Calories: 190*
- *Carbohydrates: 45g*
- *Fiber: 9g*
- *Protein: 5g*
- *Fat: 1g*

RECIPE 25: MANGO PINEAPPLE PARADISE

INGREDIENTS

1. 1 cup diced mango
2. 1 cup chopped pineapple
3. 1/2 cup coconut milk
4. 1 tablespoon honey or maple syrup (optional)
5. 1/2 teaspoon grated fresh ginger
6. Ice cubes

INSTRUCTIONS

1. Blend mango, pineapple, coconut milk, honey/maple syrup, and grated ginger until smooth.
2. Add ice cubes for a refreshing chill.
3. Pour into a glass and indulge in this taste of paradise!

NUTRITION PER SERVING

- ❖ *Calories: 220*
- ❖ *Carbohydrates: 50g*
- ❖ *Fiber: 6g*
- ❖ *Protein: 3g*
- ❖ *Fat: 5g*

RECIPE 26: PAPAYA PASSION SPLASH

INGREDIENTS

1. 1 ripe papaya, peeled and cubed
2. Pulp from 2 passionfruits
3. 1/2 cup unsweetened almond milk
4. 1 tablespoon flaxseeds
5. Splash of lime juice
6. Ice cubes

INSTRUCTIONS

1. Blend papaya, passionfruit pulp, almond milk, flaxseeds, and lime juice until creamy.
2. Incorporate ice cubes for a cooler texture.
3. Serve in a glass and relish this tropical splash!

NUTRITION PER SERVING

- ❖ *Calories: 180*
- ❖ *Carbohydrates: 35g*
- ❖ *Fiber: 9g*
- ❖ *Protein: 4g*
- ❖ *Fat: 4g*

RECIPE 27: COCONUT BANANA BREEZE

INGREDIENTS

1. 1 ripe banana
2. 1/2 cup coconut water
3. 1/2 cup pineapple chunks
4. 2 tablespoons shredded coconut
5. Handful of baby spinach
6. Ice cubes

INSTRUCTIONS

1. Blend banana, coconut water, pineapple chunks, shredded coconut, and baby spinach until smooth.
2. Add ice cubes for a cooler sensation.
3. Pour into a glass and savor this breezy tropical delight!

NUTRITION PER SERVING

- ❖ *Calories: 190*
- ❖ *Carbohydrates: 40g*
- ❖ *Fiber: 6g*
- ❖ *Protein: 3g*
- ❖ *Fat: 4g*

RECIPE 28: KIWI PAPAYA REFRESHER

INGREDIENTS

1. 2 ripe kiwis, peeled and sliced
2. 1/2 ripe papaya, seeded and cubed
3. 1/2 cup orange juice
4. 1/2 cup coconut milk
5. Ice cubes

INSTRUCTIONS

1. Blend kiwis, papaya, orange juice, and coconut milk until creamy.
2. Incorporate ice cubes for a chilled, smooth texture.
3. Pour into a glass and enjoy this refreshing tropical refresher!

NUTRITION PER SERVING

- ❖ *Calories: 200*
- ❖ *Carbohydrates: 35g*
- ❖ *Fiber: 7g*
- ❖ *Protein: 4g*
- ❖ *Fat: 5g*

RECIPE 29: ORANGE MANGO TANGO

INGREDIENTS

1. 1 cup diced mango
2. Juice from 2 oranges
3. 1/2 cup Greek yogurt (or dairy-free yogurt)
4. 1 tablespoon honey or agave syrup (optional)
5. 1/2 teaspoon turmeric (optional)
6. Ice cubes

INSTRUCTIONS

1. Blend diced mango, orange juice, Greek yogurt, honey/agave syrup, and turmeric until smooth.
2. Add ice cubes for a cool, refreshing twist.
3. Pour into a glass and revel in this vibrant, tangy tango!

NUTRITION PER SERVING

- ❖ *Calories: 220*
- ❖ *Carbohydrates: 45g*
- ❖ *Fiber: 5g*
- ❖ *Protein: 8g*
- ❖ *Fat: 3g*

RECIPE 30: PINEAPPLE COCONUT SERENITY

INGREDIENTS

1. 1 cup chopped pineapple
2. 1/2 cup coconut milk
3. 1/2 cup unsweetened almond milk
4. 1 tablespoon shredded coconut
5. 1 teaspoon vanilla extract
6. Ice cubes

INSTRUCTIONS

1. Blend chopped pineapple, coconut milk, almond milk, shredded coconut, and vanilla extract until creamy.
2. Incorporate ice cubes for a frosty texture.
3. Serve in a glass and bask in this serene tropical blend!

NUTRITION PER SERVING

- *Calories: 180*
- *Carbohydrates: 30g*
- *Fiber: 6g*
- *Protein: 2g*
- *Fat: 7g*

Conclusion

As we conclude our exploration of "Alkaline Remedies Against Cancer: Quick and Easy 30 Nourishing Plant-Based Smoothies for Cancer Prevention," we've set out on a delectable adventure that combines the bounty of nature with an effective health plan.

As we delve into the rich realm of nutrients that promote an alkaline environment inside our bodies, we have discovered the possibility of pH balance in inhibiting the progression of cancer. Every smoothie recipe, from exotic fruits to leafy greens, is designed to energize and nurture the body and soul at the same time.

These plant-based elixirs are more than just drinks; they represent a proactive move in the direction of health, using the abundance of natural components to strengthen our resistance to the development of cancer. They are an ode to flavor, a representation of sustenance, and an example of how science and culinary creativity can coexist.

May these thirty dishes serve as a tasty compass that points us in the direction of well-being as we say goodbye. Let us persist in relishing the pleasures of good health, accepting every drink as an affirmation of fortitude, a dedication to energy, and an oath to treasure the gift of life.

Please scan the QR code to access the meal plan

Date........./......./.........

Recipe Title:

ingredient

note

Description

prep time: cook time:

MY WEEKLY *Meal* Plan WEEK:

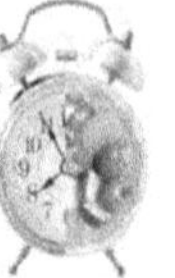

MEAL SCHEDULE

SNACKS

DRINKS

VITAMINS

FRUITS&VEGETABLES

Date........./......./.........

Recipe Title:

ingredient

note

Description

prep time: cook time:

MY WEEKLY *Meal* Plan WEEK:

MEAL SCHEDULE

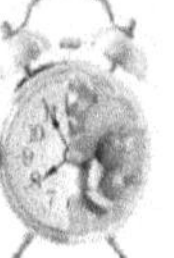

SNACKS

DRINKS

VITAMINS

FRUITS&VEGETABLES

MY WEEKLY *Meal* Plan WEEK:

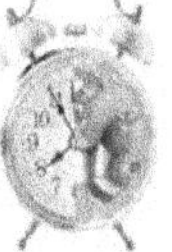

MEAL SCHEDULE

SNACKS

DRINKS

VITAMINS

FRUITS&VEGETABLES

www.ingramcontent.com/pod-product-compliance
Lightning Source LLC
Chambersburg PA
CBHW071101260726

48661CB00006B/2394